COGNITIVE BEHAVIORAL THERAPY

A CBT Beginners Guide to Defeating Anxiety, Depression, Phobias and Low-Self Esteem

S.E. Charles

DEDICATION

This book is dedicated to those in search of essential information and practical skills to help manage and control their struggle with anxiety, depression and phobias using CBT

CONTENTS

INTRODUCTION

Cognitive behavioral therapy (CBT) is a form of talking therapy which can be used to treat people with a wide range of mental health problems.

CBT is based on the idea that how we think (cognition), how we feel (emotion) and how we act (behavior) all interact together. Specifically, our thoughts determine our feelings and our behavior.

Therefore, negative and unrealistic thoughts can cause us distress and result in problems. When a person suffers with psychological distress, the way in which they interpret situations becomes skewed, which in turn has a negative impact on the actions they take.

CBT aims to help people become aware of when they make negative interpretations, and of behavioral patterns which reinforce the distorted thinking. Cognitive therapy helps people to develop alternative ways of thinking and behaving which aims to reduce their psychological distress.

In this insightful guide, you will learn useful techniques, essential information and practical skills to help you manage and control your struggle with anxiety, depression and and other mental issues using CBT

CHAPTER 1 – UNDERSTANDING THE FUNDAMENTALS

Cognitive behavioral therapy (CBT) is a form of talk therapy or psychotherapy that aims to help patients manage or control problems by altering how they think and behave. It offers a practical approach to dealing with issues.

The treatment combines the principles of both behavioral and cognitive psychology. It helps with a wide range of mental health challenges.

History of Cognitive Behavioral Therapy

Certain aspects of this form of psychotherapy have been traced back to ancient times. They are believed to have link to some ancient philosophical traditions, especially Stoicism.

Epictetus and some other Stoic philosophers thought that false beliefs that brought about unhelpful emotions can be identified and dealt with through the use of logic. Such views provided foundation for modern cognitive-behavioral theories.

The origin of CBT as we now know it is traced to the early 20th century when behavior therapy emerged. Cognitive therapy was developed in the 1960s. The two therapies were reportedly combined by psychiatrist Aaron Beck in the 1960s, leading to emergence of cognitive behavioral therapy.

The psychotherapy form was originally used for treatment of depression. While cognitive therapy is only a part of it, CBT is now often seen as incorporating all forms of cognitive-based psychotherapies.

Some Assumptions of Cognitive Behavioral Therapy

The aim with CBT is to improve the awareness of a patient when he or she is interpreting things or situations wrongly. It teaches them to be more aware of certain behaviors that can add force to negative thoughts.

A number of assumptions are involved in this treatment. They include:

• A disorder is the result of poor or wrong perception about oneself, other people, or the world. This may be caused by cognitive distortions (too much emphasis on negatives and less on positives).

• How a person views the world conditions how he or she interacts with it. There may be disordered thoughts and behaviors when this mental representation of the world is faulty.

• Symptoms of an issue can be improved by showing patients how to cope and equipping them with skills that enable them to process information rightly.

Cognitive behavioral therapy, therefore, seeks to correct cognitive distortions. It aims to fix erroneous perception and the magnification of negatives. It helps patients to see things more for what they truly are.

CBT Uses

Cognitive behavioral therapy is almost exclusively used for treatment of disorders that has connection to mental health. It has been shown to be effective for the following disorders, among others.

Anxiety disorders

There is evidence that people suffering from anxiety disorders, especially adults, can benefit from undergoing CBT. One of the techniques that therapists use for combating anxiety is exposure. The idea behind this is that people may get to unlearn fear by being exposed to the stimulus responsible for their fears.

For instance, a person who gets anxious when in a public setting may be encouraged to give a speech in front of an audience.

Eating Disorders

It is believed that cognitive behavioral therapy may be more effective for combating eating disorders. This is in comparison to the use of medications or dependence on regular talk therapy alone.

This is actually the first-line intervention for bulimia nervosa and non-specific eating disorders. Therapists can help patients to learn how to control unhelpful behaviors and avoid negative self-image and its effects.

Depression

Treatment of this disorder was one of the first uses of cognitive behavioral therapy. There is significant evidence that it is helpful for clinical depression. The therapy helps to correct the bias towards negative thoughts in depressed individuals.

Along with interpersonal psychotherapy, it is the treatment that is most efficacious for major depressive disorder, according to the American Psychiatric Association Practice Guidelines (April 2000).

Other issues that cognitive behavioral therapy may help with include:

- Psychosis
- Schizophrenia
- Smoking
- Gambling addiction
- Chronic low back pain
- Panic attacks
- Phobias
- Anger
- Chronic fatigue syndrome
- Substance abuse
- Obsessive-compulsive disorder
- Suicidal behaviors

However, people who tend to benefit the most are those who realize they have a problem that needs to be dealt with and who are open to CBT concepts and requirements. This is because the therapy depends greatly on having specific goals.

CBT works best as a short-term solution. It may not be enough in situations where the issue in focus is long-term and significantly disabling.

Types of CBT

Although cognitive behavioral therapy is only a form of psychotherapy, it is of different kinds as well. The diverse types include the following:

Cognitive emotional behavioral therapy (CEBT) - This aims to promote recovery of patients by helping them to better understand and put up with emotions. It represents a combination of certain elements of dialectical behavioral therapy and CBT.

CEBT has been used primarily with individuals suffering from eating disorders, as it offers an alternative when standard CBT is unsuccessful in relieving symptoms. Research indicates that CEBT may help reduce emotional eating, depression, and anxiety and also improve self-esteem. CEBT was developed in 2006 by British psychologist Emma Gray (née Corstorphine). Its key components include psychological education; techniques to enhance awareness of emotions and motivation to change; and strategies to restructure beliefs about the experience and expression of emotions.

Although (CEBT) was initially developed to help individuals suffering from eating disorders, its effectiveness in helping people to better understand and manage their emotions has meant that it is increasingly being used by psychologists as a 'pretreatment' to prepare patients for the process of therapy for a range of problems including anxiety, depression, obsessive compulsive disorder (OCD), and post-traumatic stress disorder (PTSD), which can often be emotionally challenging.

Brief cognitive behavioral therapy (BCBT) - Originally developed by David Rudd for soldiers in active duty abroad, this form of CBT is intended for situations where time is a constraint. The treatment is designed in such a manner that it can be completed in two sessions. Its principal aim is to prevent suicide that may result from mental health disorders.

BCBT is particularly useful in a primary care setting for patients with anxiety and depression associated with a medical condition. Because these individuals often face acute rather than chronic mental health issues and have many coping strategies already in place, BCBT can be used to enhance adjustment. Issues that may be addressed in primary care with BCBT include, but are not limited to, diet, exercise, medication compliance, mental health issues associated with a medical condition, and coping with a chronic illness or new diagnosis.

Moral Reconation Therapy (MRT) - This is a systematic approach for correction of recidivism, a propensity to repeat an unacceptable or undesirable behavior. It is typically used for felons with antisocial personality disorder (ASPD). It is now a widely accepted cognitive-behavioral approach that treats substance use disorders, trauma, domestic violence, and more.

Similar to Cognitive Behavioral Therapy (CBT), MRT aims to change thought processes and decision-making associated with addiction and criminal behavior. It utilizes a combination of psychological practices to assist with egocentric behaviors and improve moral reasoning and positive identity. MRT takes place in a group setting.

Unified Protocol and stress inoculation training are two of the other remaining types of CBT.

How to Access CBT

The typical approach to getting cognitive behavioral therapy involves going to a therapist. The treatment is provided in face-to-face sessions, each of which may last up to an hour. The number of sessions that are commonly required can range from about six to 18 sessions. The sessions usually hold 1-3 weeks apart.

Aside the traditional visits to a therapist's office, CBT is now being offered through the use of modern technology. The treatment can be provided via a computer or the internet. This is called computerized cognitive behavioral therapy (CCBT) or internet-delivered cognitive behavioral therapy (ICBT). This approach is believed to have the potential of improving access to treatment for patients. It is cheaper and more convenient.

Another method for accessing CBT is participation in group courses. You may also benefit from reading self-help materials.

How is CBT Different from Other Therapies?

Although people often refer to it as talk therapy, CBT is different from the regular types. It takes a more structured approach to treatment. Unlike in other psychotherapies, you don't just talk about anything that comes to mind. You need to be able to state your problems and the goals you wish to attain from treatment.

These set the tone for topics for discussion during any session between you and the therapist.

CBT also makes it easier for patients to have a freer relationship with their therapist. The focus is more on an equal, practical relationship rather than one where you rely entirely on the therapist to get things done. In CBT, it is common for therapists to request for feedback from patients on what they think about what's happening.

Cognitive behavioral therapy can be quite helpful when battling with cognitive distortions or excessive focus on and magnification of negative things. It assists in challenging such undesirable distortions while teaching you coping skills. Research also backs it efficiency.other underlying medical conditions by running tests for them. Effects of drug use would also be evaluated. Your doctor may suggest you see a mental health professional, such as a psychiatrist or a psychologist, if he is not able to detect the physical cause of the problem.

A mental health specialist can work with you to design the best treatment plan for your anxiety disorder, if you are found to have it. Treatment usually involves the use of medications and/or psychotherapy, the so-called "talk therapy."

There are a number of other things you can also do on your own to promote rapid improvement.

CHAPTER 2 – HOW DOES COGNITIVE BEHAVIORAL THERAPY (CBT) WORK?

Cognitive behavioral therapy (CBT) is a popular approach for combating a wide range of mental disorders, including anxiety, depression and phobias. It is a practical, goal-focused form of psychotherapy that helps patients to understand and have better control over their thoughts and feelings.

You are probably wondering how CBT, a typically short-term treatment, works? How exactly does it seek to improve the condition of patients? We discuss all you need to know in this article.

Automatic Negative Thoughts (ANTs)

A major focus in CBT is automatic negative thoughts. Renowned psychiatrist Aaron Beck is credited for inventing the term "automatic thoughts." He used it to describe thoughts that may crop up in a person's mind without them necessarily paying much attention to it, even when they have effects on their behavior.

Cognitive behavioral therapy works on a theory that what people experience isn't the main problem. The issue lies more in the interpretations they give to such events. When thoughts become negative, it becomes hard for a person to see things for what they really are.

Beck thought that these negative thoughts start during childhood. They become constant and automatic as years pass by if nothing is done to tackle them. Their intensity has the potential to become stronger.

For instance, a person who feels anxious or uncomfortable at work might have untrue negative thoughts that make them dread going to work. These unhelpful thinking patterns may cause him or her to miss work. And rather than being relieved by choosing to remain at home, the person may start regretting that decision.

CBT works to help patients deal with these automatic negative thoughts. It seeks to help people have a more realistic and objective view of situations.

In What Ways Does CBT Help?

Cognitive behavioral therapy is a practical, problem-solving approach for dealing with disorders that have connection to your mental state. There are different perspectives on how CBT works.

Cognitive behavioral therapy helps to refute beliefs that may cause you to think or act in a certain inapt way. The process starts identifying such beliefs. The patient is then encouraged to challenge these.

For instance, a person with low self-esteem sees himself or herself lesser or inferior to others. A therapist can help such a person to challenge these negative perceptions. He helps such to not see themselves as being defined by their flaws. Rather, they should consider themselves normal human beings just like other people.

CBT is probably most helpful to patients with regard to how it teaches such how to deal with thorny situations. There are diverse techniques that a therapist may adopt, depending on individual cases.

A common approach for helping patients cope is exposure, such as among people battling with anxiety. The same reasoning behind Emerson's famous quote on doing what one is afraid of also influences this.

A person suffering from anxiety will be encouraged to face their fears rather than running from them. The hope is that this will help such realize that there is nothing to be afraid of.

A person with inhibition about relating with other people may learn how to disprove certain assumptions that may be responsible. A depressed individual can learn how to control and assess their thinking patterns more realistically.

With CBT, patients can get inspiration to make certain changes that can make their lives better. Someone who lacks courage to change jobs, for instance, can feel inspired to take the step.

The collaborative approach to CBT also makes it helpful to patients. Clients don't just have to see a therapist as a know-all. Patients are encouraged to freely say whatever is on their mind. The feedbacks are then used to improve treatment as appropriate.

What is the Therapy Like?

CBT takes a structured approach. Every session between a therapist and patient follows a structure, which is developed at the beginning of a therapy. The specific problems and goals of individual patient will determine this structure.

Treatment typically begins with getting more familiar with the problems. The therapist works with a patient to identify the wrong beliefs that may be fueling negative thoughts and maladaptive behaviors. This is referred to functional analysis and helps with self-discovery, which is crucial for effective treatment.

After identifying the erroneous beliefs, a therapist then helps a patient to address the maladaptive behaviors. It is at this stage that you are taught skills that can be useful for fighting negative thoughts and controlling how they impact your behavior.

Both your therapist and you will decide on topics to address at the beginning of each session. The problems and goals identified earlier will provide the basis for a topic. This sort of planning also makes it possible to briefly go over conclusion from an earlier session.

Homework is an integral part of CBT. You should expect to be assigned tasks that you are to do at home. Your doctor will expect you to come with a report of how you did this when next you'll be meeting.

Importance of Homework

The homework your therapist will give between sessions often involves some level of self-analysis. You should expect to spend time evaluating your thoughts and feelings. This may not necessarily be an easy thing to do and some patients may fail to do such homework.

However, at-home assignments are very important in ensuring you get the most out of CBT. Experts say people who are open to doing these tend to have better results.

A sample assignment at the start may be to keep a record of events or situations that make you feel anxious or depressed.

Homework later in the treatment will involve doing things that can help you deal with a problem. If you are suffering from depression, for instance, you may be encouraged to spend time with a friend before the next session with your therapist.

How Helpful is CBT?

Cognitive behavioral therapy is one of the most-researched forms of psychotherapy. When it comes to managing psychological disorders, it represents a potentially more helpful approach than the use of drugs. It compares very well to medications for treatment of anxiety disorders and depression in the short-term.

CBT effects last longer and may reduce your reliance on drugs for managing a particular disorder. There is lower risk of relapse unlike what obtains with the use of medications. Research suggests that a 12-session therapy offers similar benefits as using drugs for a period of two years for treatment of depression.

This longer-lasting effect is a reason why there is increasing interest in CBT.

However, this treatment will not work equally well for everybody. Those who benefit the most are people who are open, persistent and ready to devote time and effort to it. This therapy is not ideal for people who expect so much in so little time. Some may have to devote a period of time longer than usual to the treatment.

Essentially, CBT is more suitable for individuals who are well at home with psychotherapy that takes a structured, goal-focused approach. It is for people who are ready to cooperate effectively with a therapist.

The expertise of a particular therapist also matters.

CBT is Evolving

Cognitive behavioral therapy continues to evolve. Researchers are still learning about how it can be more helpful to people, especially those with tough problems. New ideas and techniques are on the horizon.

The therapy isn't based on entirely new principles. Some underlying concepts have been known for at least about 2,000 years and well proven to work. CBT may be seen as providing a reminder of what people already know. It basically helps you to put helpful principles into use, not just to know about them.

Talk to your doctor or check out the directory on the website of the National Association of Cognitive Behavioral Therapists if you wish to find a certified therapist in your area.

S.E. Charles

CHAPTER 3 - USING COGNITIVE BEHAVIORAL THERAPY (CBT) FOR ANXIETY

Anxiety disorders are among a variety of psychological disorders that cognitive behavioral therapy (CBT) is thought to help with. There's actually research evidence showing that this treatment can be beneficial.

A qualified CBT therapist is able to provide you with information and skills that can help you overcome your anxiety. He or she teaches you skills for dealing with your problem. You get to learn how to think in a more realistic manner.

Treating Anxiety with CBT

There are different classes of drugs that anyone can use for battling anxiety. The level of efficiency of each one differs. But what medications seem to have more in common is the potential for side effects.

Cognitive behavioral therapy offers a safer method of

treating mental disorders, especially the less severe forms. It doesn't come with the kinds of side effects that typically accompany medicines.

However, the appeal of CBT isn't just the safety. It is considered as the best option for some people suffering from anxiety disorders. The treatment doesn't just treat the symptoms, unlike drugs. It seeks to deal with the underlying causes of a disorder.

In addition to helping to unravel the underlying causes, CBT equips you with skills to have better control over your anxiety.

This form of psychotherapy is the most popular for treatment of anxiety disorders. It is a combination of both cognitive therapy and behavior therapy.

The cognitive part takes notice of how cognition distortions or negative thoughts fuel anxiety. On the other hand, behavior therapy deals with your reaction to these thoughts or how they impact your behavior.

This essentially means CBT views your anxiety as the result of your thinking patterns, not external events. It, therefore, seeks to rectify how you view yourself and the world around you.

Studies have shown that people with anxiety issues can benefit from CBT. Alone, its efficacy is comparable to that of psychoactive drugs for treatment of less severe forms of anxiety, depression and eating disorders, among others.

CBT has been well shown to be helpful to adult patients with anxiety disorders. It is one of only two psychosocial therapies that psychiatry residents must be trained in.

Dealing with Negative Thoughts

CBT takes a systematic approach to helping you deal with negative thoughts and, so, have better control of your anxiety. The technique used is called cognitive restructuring or cognitive reframing. It involves you challenging negative thoughts that make you feel anxious.

There are three basic steps involved in the cognitive restructuring process. They are:

Identification – Your therapist works with you to identify maladaptive or irrational thinking patterns and beliefs. A person with anxiety issue typically considers situations to be more hazardous than they really are. You can identify these by paying closer attention to what you think about when feeling anxious.

Dispute – After identifying these negative thoughts, you are then encouraged to challenge them. You will be taught how to question the veracity of your thinking patterns. If you fear that something bad might happen in a situation, for instance, your therapist can teach how to realistically assess the probability of such happening.

Alteration – Cognitive restructuring also involves altering or replacing negative, fear-inducing thoughts. This should be easier after completing the first two steps successfully. Once you are able to prove that your anxious thoughts are irrational, your therapist helps you to replace them with positive, more realistic ones. This step may also involve the use of self-affirmations when in a situation that induces anxiety.

In Vivo Exposure

A crucial element of cognitive behavioral therapy when it comes to combating anxiety is exposure. This is called in vivo exposure therapy or simply exposure therapy. It works on the long-held belief that the death of fear is certain when people confront their fears.

It is not uncommon for people to avoid situations that induce their anxiety. For example, a person with social anxiety disorder will avoid situations where they have to be in a crowd. It gets worse if they think they will be the center of attention.

But in vivo exposure turns things on its head. This technique exposes you to that very thing you fear. The belief here is that doing this will enable you to overcome such fears.

For example, if you dread public speaking, your therapist may give you exercises that entail giving a speech.

Exposure to anxiety-inducing situations might sound counterintuitive and capable of worsening the problem. But when you are repeatedly exposed to things that scare you there is evidence that your fear can subside. This much has actually been known for thousands of years.

It should be noted, though, that you are not just told to confront your fears sort of no holds barred. In vivo exposure takes a systematic approach. Your therapist starts at a level that is more bearable for you and then progress from there. This is referred to as systematic desensitization.

You may likely be given a list of actions that you are to take gradually until you are able to overcome your fears.

Exposure doesn't necessarily mean being in an anxious situation; you may be asked to imagine such.

Other CBT Skills for Fighting Anxiety

We have discussed how cognitive behavioral therapy can be helpful for treating anxiety by teaching you certain skills. It helps you to be aware when having thought distortions or when you are ruminating. It equips you with skills for dispelling negative thoughts.

Furthermore, you may also learn the following through CBT:

Self-kindness

Self-criticism is a major contributor to anxiety, especially among people with social anxiety disorder. You judge yourself harshly over what you think are imperfections. You fear that one of these seeming imperfections may rare its ugly head and embarrass you.

With CBT, you can learn to be kinder to yourself. You can get to know how to prove such unkind thoughts wrong or to question their genuineness. The therapy may help you to be more aware that whatever flaw doesn't define the real, complete you.

Managing uncertainty

People who suffer from anxiety or depression have been known to exhibit intolerance of uncertainty. This contributes to and worsens the disorder.

An anxious person is usually in double mind or unsure about the likelihood of what they fear happening. He or she is not entirely certain a negative event will not happen.

This causes such a person to procrastinate, check excessively for signs of danger, or to avoid taking an action altogether.

CBT can equip you with skills for overcoming such uncertainty.

Better mind control

Cognitive behavioral therapy can teach you how to have firmer control over your thought process. You get to learn how to take advantage of mindfulness techniques to enhance both your mental and physical health.

By practicing mindfulness, you may find it easier coping with your anxiety. It will help you to reduce how much or often you ruminate. It can also enhance your ability to take the right decisions whenever you are beginning to feel anxious.

CBT can be an effective weapon in your arsenal for combating anxiety. It is important to note, however, that it is not a quick fix. You should be willing to cooperate with your therapist and give the process time to get maximum benefits.

CHAPTER 4- USING COGNITIVE BEHAVIORAL THERAPY (CBT) FOR DEPRESSION

Cognitive behavioral therapy is a form of psychotherapy that combines elements of both cognitive and behavioral therapies. It is a very popular type of psychological therapy. The treatment is proven to be effective for a wide array of disorders, among which is depression.

It works on a person's thinking patterns, which are the core of problem in mental disorders. The efficacy is similar to, possibly even better than, that of medications. In this chapter we learn more about how CBT can be beneficial for dealing with depression.

What's Depression Like?

It's not totally unusual to hear people say "I'm feeling

depressed." But that doesn't mean the same thing for everyone who makes such a statement.

Some feel miserable or sad for a short while as a result of some events in their lives, such as the loss of a loved one. They soon get better and move on with life. This is not the case with anyone suffering from clinical depression.

A common feature of this mental health disorder is a feeling of sadness that just won't go away. Low mood usually results in depressed individuals withdrawing from social activities and relationships. At its worst, the condition may cause you to feel helpless, worthless and hopeless.

Depression disrupts the normal functioning of your brain. You are always having negative thoughts. The disorder makes you to place more emphasis on the negatives than the positives in your life. It causes mental fog, concentration issues and memory problems.

The effects of depression don't stop at the psychological level. They can also reflect on general body functions. You may experience loss of appetite and low libido as a result. The disorder can cause sleep disruptions and fatigue, among other issues.

How Does CBT Work for Depression?

Cognitive behavioral therapists view mental disorders such as depression as a result of thought distortions and maladaptive behaviors. They usually do not consider a problem the result of personality traits, but rather the effect of your views or beliefs. The attempt in therapy is to work on the latter.

Core beliefs – These are the assumptions that you hold and which influence how you view the world and yourself. A depressed person becomes so accustomed to negative core beliefs that he or she no longer disputes them. For instance, a person might think, "I am useless," and will not able to question that assertion at all.

Intermediate beliefs – These are a branch of core beliefs but are different. Intermediate beliefs incorporate attitudes rules and assumptions. They influence your perception of situation by provoking "automatic thoughts," which are involuntary thoughts or images in your mind. A good example may be thinking people don't like you because they didn't sit close to you at a public gathering.

Seeing their relationship to intermediate beliefs, core beliefs can cause or worsen depression when they are dysfunctional. They give room to dysfunctional rules and negative automatic thoughts.

The aim in CBT is to help you identify erroneous core beliefs or cognitive distortions that can influence your behavior. The treatment helps patients to alter dysfunctional negative core beliefs they hold about themselves.

Your therapist helps you to be aware of these thoughts. He then shows you how you can replace them with positive thoughts. This will often involve the use of self-affirmations.

For instance, for those times you think or say, "I am worthless," you may be encouraged to challenge that by telling yourself something like, "That's not true. I have a lot to offer the people around me."

What to Expect in Treatment

Cognitive behavioral therapy is usually offered in a one-on-one setting, although you can also get it in a group setting or by reading self-help materials. It is ideally supervised by a professional trained in mental treatment techniques, especially in CBT.

Treatment is done in sessions, with each one lasting up to an hour. It is typically short-term and takes place in 10 to 20 sessions in most cases. Duration of treatment may be shorter or may extend beyond a year, depending on the severity of your depression.

Your therapist will collaborate with you to establish treatment goals at the beginning. This will inform what to do during each session.

There will be less focus on your personality trait or your past. Emphasis will be more on your current thinking patterns and behaviors with a view to changing them. This clearly sets CBT apart from psychoanalysis, which seeks to find the root of a problem in the past.

You should expect to be given assignments to do at home between sessions. Before the end of treatment, your therapist will teach you skills that can be useful for keeping depression from coming back.

How Effective is CBT for Depression?

Cognitive behavioral therapy is well-documented to be effective for dealing with a variety of psychological disorders. There isn't any other form of psychotherapy that has as much evidence of effectiveness as this one.

This is mainly because researchers find it easier to study than the other ones.

There is evidence that CBT works as well as some medications that are used for treatment of depression. Research suggests that people who get the therapy may be up to about 50 percent less likely to suffer a recurrence of depression within a year, compared to those who take only medications.

But you shouldn't take this to mean that CBT is a perfect substitute for antidepressants. While it may be enough to deal with some mild or moderate cases, the therapy will most likely not suffice for severe depression.

People who have severe forms of the disorder should see this psychotherapy as a complementary treatment. It can help their condition to improve faster, with the treatment effects also lasting longer, when combined with medications.

What are the Risks?

A major reason more people seem to be embracing CBT is that it is safer when compared to drugs. You will often see people describe it as being free of side effects.

However, the therapy is not entirely devoid of discomfort, specifically of the emotional nature. This is because it often involves encouraging patients to confront things or situations they fear.

For instance, you may be asked to face up to the reality of the loss of a loved one that might be responsible for your depression. This is not an easy thing to do. But the aim is to help you master the unhelpful, painful thoughts such an event might be causing.

Cognitive behavioral therapy is a well-proven means of beating depression and other anxiety disorders. It works as well as medications, or even better, for some people.

This treatment is especially useful and most effective for treating mild or moderate cases. If you can find yourself a therapist with the right expertise, it can help with severe form of depression as well. The efficacy improves greatly when used in combination with antidepressants and other drugs for treating the disorder.

It is important to state that you should not stop taking your drugs when starting CBT. You should speak to your doctor first before quitting. This also applies when working with an experienced therapist. Stopping your medications may aggravate the disorder and you will feel worse for it.

CHAPTER 5 – OTHER CONDITIONS TREATED BY CBT

Cognitive behavioral therapy (CBT) is a psychosocial intervention for improving mental health. It teaches patients how to stay in control of their thought patterns and have a more enjoyable life.

The treatment was originally designed for dealing with depression. But its use was expanded to several other mental health issues, including anxiety. Today, many people know CBT as being for control of depression and anxiety. In this lesson, we discuss some other conditions that it can help with.

Eating Disorders

There are many approaches available for treating eating disorders, but CBT is arguably the best. Researchers have found that it is more reliable and efficacious than drugs and interpersonal psychotherapy alone. It was originally used as a tool for fighting bulimia nervosa, but its uses have now extended to other eating disorders as well.

The treatment aims to combat eating disorders by dealing with negative thoughts pertaining to body shape, weight or size. It helps to rein in thoughts capable of encouraging risky compensatory behaviors.

CBT is the first-line treatment for bulimia nervosa. Research shows that it is the best approach for combating the condition. Treatment of this eating disorder and others commonly involves the use of a type of CBT known as CBT-Enhanced (CBT-E).

Obsessive-Compulsive Disorder (OCD)

OCD is a mental health disorder that causes a person to have recurring, undesirable thoughts (obsessions) and to check things or perform some tasks repeatedly (compulsions). An individual with this disorder has no control over these obsessions and compulsions.

CBT is considered probably the best treatment for fighting this disorder. In this case, it mainly involves the use of two techniques, namely: cognitive therapy (CT) and exposure and response prevention (ERP) therapy.

In cognitive therapy, the belief is that there are certain negative thoughts driving OCD. A therapist, therefore, helps you to identify and control thinking patterns that are responsible for anxiety, distress or unusual behavior. You get to learn how to be aware when your brain is sending wrong signals and how to control your response to such.

The ERP technique involves exposing you to situations or things that trigger your obsessions and compulsions. The aim here is to modify your response to such and so improve your condition. This exposure is done gradually in a controlled setting.

CBT is the form of psychotherapy with the strongest evidence of helping people with OCD.

Bipolar Disorder

There is evidence that people suffering from bipolar disorder may benefit from CBT. This condition, which used to be known as manic depression, causes extreme and abnormal shifts or swings in mood, from mania to depression.

Research has shown that the thinking patterns of patients have effect on the mood swings seen in bipolar disorder cases. For example, researchers found in a 2015 study in the journal Psychology and Psychotherapy (formerly the British Journal of Medical Psychology) that very negative thoughts can give rise to what they called "descent behaviors," such as seen in depression. On the other hand, highly positive thoughts can result in "ascent behaviors," the likes associated with mania.

CBT teaches bipolar patients techniques that they can use to prevent their thoughts driving them to either extremes of mood. An important aspect is cognitive reframing, which helps to identify, challenge and replace negative or distorted thoughts.

Bipolar disorder was among conditions that were reported to improve with this therapy in a review by the INSERM Collective Expertise Centre.

Sleep Problems

Do you find it difficult getting quality sleep? Cognitive

behavioral therapy may be the solution you're looking for. It is more likely to be beneficial if you are middle-aged or older.

Insomnia is a common disorder. It affects millions of people every year. The condition makes it difficult to fall or stay asleep or causes you wake too early and unable to go back to sleep.

Cognitive behavioral therapy for insomnia, also referred to as CBT-I, is often a first-line intervention for sleep problems. An idea behind this structured treatment program is that your thoughts are responsible for your inability to get quality bedtime.

Your therapist helps you to identify problematic thoughts and behaviors - this may require you keeping a sleep diary. He teaches you how to get rid of or manage these. You also get to learn about good habits that can help you to sleep better.

CBT for sleep problems may be better than sleeping pills. It does more than just relieving symptoms; it helps to address the underlying causes.

Chronic Pain

Pain is something many of us have become used to. Estimate has it that some 100 million people in the United States battle with chronic pain, the type that extends beyond 12 weeks. This obviously explains why the use of painkillers is so common.

Chronic pain is not easy to deal with. This is because it

may no longer be an indication of an underlying problem. People often continue to feel it even after the original cause has been dealt with.

CBT is said to be a great nonmedical approach to tackling this type of pain. It can be used alone or together with other treatment options. The therapy is recognition of how pain is the result of processes taking place in your brain.

CBT helps to counter or reverse your reactions to chronic pain. For example, pain can result in you withdrawing from normal social activities. It may lead to fatigue, mood changes, depression, and sleep problems. It helps you to be more active and regain much of the life you've lost.

The main impediment to the use of this therapy for treatment of chronic pain is doubt. Many patients, and even care providers, don't think pain can be all in the head. This effectively nullifies considerable scientific evidence that shows CBT may help.

Schizophrenia

By the looks of it, cognitive behavioral therapy may not seem like a nice remedy for schizophrenia. But this disorder was among those that the treatment was found to be effective for in the INSERM review mentioned earlier. These are also other studies that reported similar potential.

CBT helps patients to stay in control of their thoughts. It is useful for modifying the thought patterns, emotional responses, and behaviors. This makes it potentially beneficial for regulating how a schizophrenic individual thinks, feels and behaves.

The therapy can help patients come to the realization that the issues they are having do not define them. It offers a way of improving the effects of treatment with medications. It is not uncommon for patients to continue experiencing distorted thoughts, hallucinations, paranoia, and lack of pleasure, among other symptoms, with pharmacologic therapy.

Alongside medications, the efficacy of CBT for schizophrenia has been well demonstrated over the years. It helps to deal with symptoms that remain after taking drugs.

Other Conditions

There are many other conditions or issues that CBT may be helpful for combating. One of this is smoking. Therapists will often view this as a behavior that people for coping with the stressors in life. Therefore, treatment can, for instance, involve seeking to replace smoking with better coping mechanisms.

Researchers at Stanford University School of Medicine found that CBT can be an effective tool for helping people quit smoking. They observed that people who got the therapy had an abstinence rate of 45 percent, compared to 29 percent among those who didn't, at 20 weeks.

Other conditions that may be treated with CBT include:

- Psychosis
- Gambling addiction
- Internet addiction
- Posttraumatic stress disorder (PTSD)
- Chest pain
- Chronic fatigue syndrome

- Attention deficit hyperactivity disorder (ADHD)
- Panic disorder
- Body dysmorphic disorder
- Alcohol dependency

The level of effectiveness varies among the different conditions. CBT was proven or presumed to work for these in some meta-analyses. But there are cases where some researchers found that it didn't help with some conditions it was thought useful for.

Essentially, cognitive behavioral therapy may work as well as shown in some studies or might not. You should have this in mind when seeking treatment. Also, realize that the therapy is not a quick fix.

CHAPTER 6 – FINDING THE RIGHT THERAPIST

So you are having some issues in your life and learned that therapy, especially cognitive behavioral therapy (CBT), could be helpful for overcoming them. After all, there is convincing evidence that this treatment can be helpful for a variety of conditions that have connection to the state of your mental health.

But the immediate problem you have now is finding the right therapist. You are correct to be concerned about getting this part right. It has been shown that the level of expertise of a supervising professional influences the degree of success.

The attempt here is to educate you about some important things worth knowing when finding a therapist. You will also learn about questions you should ask in the course of your search.

Conditions Treated with Therapy

There are many conditions that are today treated with

psychotherapy. Of its different forms, CBT is the most popular and the most evidence based. Therapy typically helps to address negative thoughts that may be reflecting as maladaptive or unusual behaviors.

Psychotherapy is used for dealing with psychological disorders. Anxiety and depression are the issues it is most known to be beneficial for. But beyond these two, there is a wide range of disorders that this kind of treatment is thought capable of helping with. They include:

- Panic disorder
- Low self-esteem
- Trauma
- Phobias
- Attention deficit hyperactivity disorder (ADHD)
- Obsession-compulsive disorder (OCD)
- Anger
- Chronic pain
- Eating disorders

If a problem has a connection to your thoughts or behaviors, chances are that it can improve with therapy. You can benefit from it if you have problems that have effect on your quality of life.

What Professionals Can Help?

There are many types of professionals that do offer psychotherapy. But the training, main areas of focus and experience of each one differ. Below are some of the more common professionals that provide therapy. These are typically knowledgeable about different psychotherapy techniques, including CBT.

Psychiatrists – These are among the best professionals to approach when in need of therapy. They are property trained to understand the workings of both your body and brain. Psychiatrists diagnose and treat psychiatric disorders. They are also licensed to prescribe medications.

Psychologists – These are professionals trained in the field of psychology. Psychologists, who are usually holders of doctoral degrees, are very knowledgeable about the human mind and behavior. They may help to unravel emotional issues at the base of a problem. Their main tool of trade is CBT.

Professional counselors – When properly trained and licensed, counselors can help with a wide variety of mental health issues, including addiction, depression, stress and substance abuse. They are certified or licensed to diagnose and treat psychological disorders. Professional counselors typically need to hold at least a master's degree in counseling. They also need thousands of post-master's degree experience.

Social workers – You can also seek therapists from a social worker when having relationship or personal issues. These professionals show concerns for people and help them function better wherever they find themselves.

Marriage and family therapists or family counselors may also provide therapy to people.

The best type of professionals to work with depends on the main form of psychotherapy you have in focus. But when it comes to CBT, it is best to go with therapists that are known to have specific training in it. Psychiatrists and psychologists are among the best options in this case.

Finding Therapists for Children and Adolescents

With the different kinds of professionals that provide

therapy these days, it is easy to get the choice wrong when a young child or a teenager is the one in need of treatment. Most therapists work with adults and it is rather tough finding the right one for children and teenagers.

Psychiatrists may be the best option for people in these age groups. Most other professionals who work with adults, including psychologists, may not be ideal. But it is surprising to note that the latter group is often sought for children when having mental health issues.

For instance, most children with ADHD are reportedly treated by a primary care doctor, pediatrician or professional counselor. But research shows that majority of these patients had another psychological disorder.

Psychiatrists are well trained to understand the brain and the body as well as the link between them. This makes them the most ideal for young patients, especially those battling depression.

How to Select a Therapist

The fact that how much you benefit from therapy depends, to a large extent, on the particular professional you are working with can't be overemphasized. Therefore, you want to ensure you get your choice right. Below are some tips you can work with.

Ask for recommendations

Chances are you have friends or family members who have had or know someone who had mental health issues. You can ask such if they can recommend the expert they worked with.

If you have a complete list of care providers from your managed care company, you can pass such list to your loved ones or colleagues for any recommendation. You can also share the list with your primary care doctor to see if they can recommend a good therapist from there.

You may also be able to get recommendations from a local university. The psychology or psychiatry department of such institution may know a good practicing professional that was trained there.

Go through associations

Professional associations often maintain a directory of certified members on their website. You can find a therapist through that means. It is also possible to contact the association to tell you more about a particular therapist you might have in focus.

The American Psychiatric Association and the American Psychological Association are examples of these associations. They can provide you with a list of professionals in your area.

Ask questions

When visiting a therapist for the first time, you should have a list of questions to ask. You should find out, for example, if they have training in a particular technique you have in focus. In the case of CBT, it helps for such to be certified by the National Association of Cognitive Behavioral Therapists (NACBT) and/or the Academy of Cognitive Therapy (ACT).

You should find out how long they have been in practice. Ask questions on similar cases as yours they have handled and the results. It may also help to find out if they have current litigation against them, if possible.

Some experts think it is better to work with therapists that have passed through therapy themselves. The idea here is that it is more helpful if they have experienced what it feels like. You may ask question pertaining to this.

Assess level of comfort

You should be observant of how a therapist communicates and responds to questions. Do you feel they are someone you will be comfortable working with? This is an important consideration that can greatly influence how much you benefit from therapy.

But then, this doesn't necessarily mean being overly comfortable. You just need to be sure your therapist can communicate well with and connect to you. They should listen and ask questions that can help them understand you and your issues better.

Although you may not get better overnight, therapy is very effective for getting your life back on track. It can help you to love and be kind to yourself. It helps you to find life more enjoyable and improves your chances of having a brighter future.

But the journey to the ideal starts with finding the right therapist. The ideas shared in this article should help towards that.

CHAPTER 7 – HOW TO APPLY CBT IN YOUR LIFE

It is no longer news that cognitive behavioral therapy (CBT) is a highly effective form of psychotherapy. The efficacy has been shown in both clinical and "real life" settings. Many people know it more for treatment of anxiety disorders and depression.

There are various techniques that have been developed and used in this therapy to make it suitable for different kinds of disorders. You can enjoy great mental health and wonderful life skills by applying these techniques or exercises in your life. In this chapter... we learn how.

Problem Identification and Resolution

There is a reason you feel a certain unpleasant way. There are underlying issues that can make you think and react in a certain manner. For instance, fear of criticism could be why you are afraid of speaking in the public.

CBT helps to identify problems and negative thoughts. It emphasizes the importance of thinking of ways to overcome problems after identifying them. It teaches how to be more active in challenging problems and finding solutions.

For example, CBT can cause you to take steps to mix more with people when experiencing social withdrawal or loneliness due to a mental health issue.

Thought Records

Journaling is an important aspect of CBT. It is a means of identifying the underlying causes of a problem. When having negative thoughts in your mind, you write them down. You then think of how you can deal with the particular problem bothering you.

For instance, when you think, "I am unlovable," you can write it somewhere. You then assess those things that make you feel that way – maybe it's how people talk to or behave towards you.

You don't stop at the evidence that suggests you are unlovable. The aim with thought records is to keep everything in balance, or close to. For the earlier example, you can try to back to times when someone thought you were a lovable person. You use that evidence to counter that which makes you feel unlovable.

Reframe your thought processes

When you notice that you are in a negative thought process, examine your beliefs that are coming up. If those beliefs don't make sense to you, you can simply choose to change them. Changing your perspective changes your reality.

Graded Exposure

This is a CBT technique that involves exposing yourself to the cause of your problem, stress or fear. For example, if you are the type that shies away from being in a social setting, you are exposed to that very environment. The belief is that exposure will help you to unlearn your fear.

However, this doesn't mean you are exposed to stressful situations all at once. The "graded" part suggests that this is a gradual, measured process. You are exposed to the situation you dread one step at a time. This enables you develop skills for controlling your fear.

Graded exposure works best for people with anxiety disorders or simple phobias.

Activity Scheduling

Another CBT technique that you can apply in your life is that of having set time for activities you enjoy. Activity scheduling is especially beneficial to people suffering from depression. The condition often makes such to lose interest in what they used to enjoy.

Mental health issues generally may not put you in the mood for doing things, even when such may be beneficial. You should, therefore, make conscious effort to schedule activities you enjoy, or used to, on different days of the week. An activity that gives you a sense of accomplishment can also work.

Devotion to such a schedule can help to reduce the frequency and intensity of negative thoughts.

Self-Affirmations

Self-affirmation is an important theory in social and psychological research. It offers a good means of taking more notice of and asserting the value of oneself and one's existence. You may think of it as a rebuff of any threat to the idea of self.

CBT and other forms of psychotherapy often involve the use of self-affirmations or self-statements. This is a good technique for quieting negative thoughts that may be threatening to derail your life and pleasure.

For example, when you feel like saying, "People don't like me," when someone shows no concern about you, it may be better to say something like "It's normal for some people not to be friendly towards me." This will keep you from dwelling perpetually on the negative.

In therapy, you are encouraged to write down self-affirmations that you can be using frequently.

Be Aware of Cognitive Distortions

Cognitive distortions are what many in the treatment field affectionately refer to as stinking thinking. These thought processes are not our best and lead us to more negative behaviors than positive behaviors.

Here are 10 examples of Cognitive Distortions:

• ***Black and white thinking***- may be referred as polarized thinking, not seeing the grey.

• ***Catastrophizing***- assuming the worst-case scenario, magnifying the negative and minimizing the positive.

• Overgeneralizing- assuming all experiences and people are the same, based on one negative experience.

• *Personalization*- believing that you are at least partially responsible for everything bad that happens around you.

• *Jumping to conclusions*- being convinced of something with little to no evidence to support it.

• *Fallacy of fairness*- being too concerned over whether everything is fair.

• *Control fallacies*- thinking everything that happens to you is either all your fault or not at all your fault.

• *Fallacy of change*- expecting others to change to suit your needs or desires.

• *Blaming*- pointing to others when looking for a cause of any negative event, instead of looking at yourself.

• *Always being right*- believing that it is absolutely unacceptable to be wrong.

These and other behaviors can be minimized by the practice of mindfulness. The more aware you become the more control you have over your thoughts.

Unraveling Cognitive Distortions

This is a primary goal of CBT and can be practiced with or without the help of a therapist. In order to unravel cognitive distortions, you must first become aware of the distortions from which you commonly suffer. Part of this involves identifying and challenging harmful automatic thoughts, which frequently fall into one of the 10 categories listed above.

Mindfulness and Relaxation

Psychological issues make it hard to have firm control over your mind and thoughts. They tend to go rather haywire when having any of these problems. The use of mindfulness techniques, such as meditation, as in CBT can be useful for bringing it all together. They help to dispel contemplations and cognitive distortions by bringing your attention back to the present.

Relaxation techniques that are taught in therapy is something you can put to good use in everyday life. These can make you less anxious and reduce stress. Breathing exercises are a good example. These help you have better control over your breathing to guard against anxiety. They make it easier for you to think more clearly and creatively.

Successive Approximations

This is a technique that aims to help a person to gradually exhibit a certain kind of behavior. Approximation may be described as any behavior similar to but not exactly the desired behavior. You may then see successive approximations as a series of steps to attaining a target behavior.

Essentially, if you wish to overcome a problem and behave in a better way, you should aim to achieve this gradually. It is well known that breaking a large task into smaller parts makes it less daunting to tackle.

For example, a first step might be to read about public speaking in the comfort of your home if you are someone who dreads it. You can then watch videos of people speaking eloquently before a large audience or attend such an event to assess how they do it. Then, you continue with other steps until you are finally able to speak, at least relatively, well in public.

Successive approximations apparently go together with exposure.

CBT Can Make a Big Difference in Your Life

While cognitive behavioral therapy is by no means a quick fix, it offers a proven way of overcoming mental health issues. You will find your life more enjoyable when you religiously apply its techniques or exercises in your life.

This therapy teaches you how to view life in a different way. With its aid, you will learn how to identify distorted cognitions and negative thoughts. It teaches you how to be more aware when having distressing thoughts as well as to question the validity of such.

For instance, when you feel uncomfortable or distressed, therapists encourage patients to try and write down what they are thinking at such times. This can go a long way in knowing what thoughts to watch out for to guard against episodes of anxiety or depression, for instance.

Self-love is important, but it may be difficult when having a mental health issue. By applying CBT principles, you can learn to love yourself more. You learn that you are not just all that seems to be going wrong in your life.

The therapy helps patients to realize that life is about up and downs. Sometimes you are up and at other times you are down. By applying CBT in your life, you become more aware that things going wrong are a normal part of life and not something to kill yourself over. This has the potential to make you find life more enjoyable.

You can also be more productive by putting the techniques of cognitive behavioral therapy to use in your life. They make you more mindful. Instead of bringing yourself down with things that have gone sour in your life, you try to bring yourself to the present - to things that currently demand your attention and matter.

From all of these, it is easy to see that your life can become way better and more enjoyable by applying CBT techniques.

Please Leave a Review

Finally, if you enjoyed this book, please take the time to share your thoughts and post a review. It'd be greatly appreciated!

That review and feedback will help me improve the content in my books – and make each and every one more relevant and helpful to you.

Thank you again and good luck!

S.E. Charles

S.E. Charles

Preview of 'Combating Migraines: The Essential Guide to Effectively Get Rid of Migraines' by S.E. Charles

11 Common Migraine Causes and Triggers

A migraine attack can be a very awful experience. It can strike so suddenly or build gradually. It is definitely not comforting to realize that scientists do not yet fully understand the causes.

But while the causes may not be clearly understood, scientists believe that a number of different factors can bring on an attack. We discuss some of the common possible causes or triggers in this article. Being familiar with these factors could be helpful for nipping the problem in the bud.

1. Caffeine

Coffee is a favorite of many people, especially those looking to stay alert and be more productive. Its consumption, however, exposes people to a common trigger of migraine: caffeine. Those who take several cups of coffee each day appear to suffer from attacks more.

What is rather strange here, though, is that some people report feeling better after taking a cup of coffee. Suddenly stopping intake has also been found to be a possible trigger.

Nevertheless, it may help to reduce your caffeine intake. You should note that coffee isn't the only source. You will also find it in pain relievers. It is present in chocolate as well.

2. Stress

This is a major reason why people experience this primary headache disorder. The link between stress and migraine is a very strong one. Estimate has it that it contributes to almost 7 of every 10 attacks.

Researchers observed in a study that the daily head pain experience of most patients (up to 70 percent) was connected to their daily stress level.

Again, as with caffeine, the effect of stress isn't entirely clear-cut. There are people who typically have their attacks when stress level reduces, such as on weekends. This phenomenon is referred to as "weekend headaches."

3. Environment

What happens around you, in your environment, can lead to migraine. For instance, change in altitude or humidity could bring about an attack. Increase in temperature and storms are also among changes in the environment that could set off a migraine episode.

4. Food

Your choice of food also has a possible role to play in whether you have migraine or not. Perhaps, the most common among the many types of foods that may cause you to have an attack are those that have monosodium glutamate (MSG) and histamine. Cheese and other forms of dairy products are examples.

There is a common belief that sweet foods, such as chocolate, and artificial sweeteners can trigger migraine.

However, this may not be entirely correct. Experts think cravings for sweet things are only indicative of an imminent attack.

Also, note that food consumption isn't the only problem; lack of it is also an issue. You may be at a greater risk of having migraine if you regularly skip meals.

5. Hormonal Changes

In women, changes in hormone levels can lead to migraine. The disorder seems to have close association with female hormones.

Estrogen, in particular, appears to play a role. Women with the disorder typically report having headaches around their menstrual periods when the levels of this hormone fluctuate or drop.

These hormonal imbalances worsen during menopause, a period when more women feel the pain. The hormonal factor probably explains why females tend to have migraine more than males.

6. Medications

It is possible that the drugs you use may also cause you to have migraine. Hormonal treatments that women receive, including hormone replacement therapy and oral contraceptives, may trigger or aggravate the headache. Nitroglycerin and other vasodilators can also play a role.

Furthermore, excessive use of acute medications can intensify the attacks.

7. Sensory stimuli

It is observed that both natural and artificial lights do cause some people to suffer headache. Sun glare, bright or flickering lights, or fluorescent bulbs can be a problem. This makes some patients to seek solace in a dark place.

Strong smells or odors, such as cigarette smoke or perfume, may precipitate an attack in some people. Also, loud sound or noise can trigger migraine.

8. Alcohol

People with migraine increase their risk of experiencing an attack with consumption of alcohol. Red wine, in particular, can be a problem despite some health benefits that are associated with it. It contains the amino acid tyramine, which research shows has a link to migraine.

Tyramine is not limited to red wine. Cheese and chocolate are other example of foods you will also find it in.

Note that red wine is not necessarily the worst culprit among alcoholic drinks. It just happens to be the one that researchers seem to know more about.

9. Sleep

The quality of bedtime you get can be a factor in migraine attacks. This is easy to understand when you consider how sleep fights stress and refreshes the body.

You may be at an increased risk of severe headache when you sleep too little or maintain an irregular sleep routine. Some people report having migraine when they sleep too late in the night or find it difficult to.

Things can even get worse when poor or irregular bed schedule results in headaches. The pain keeps you up for a significant part of the night. This increases your risk of having a sleep disorder, which aggravates the migraine.

While too little sleep is bad, too much is not any better. People sometimes report having headache when sleeping or dozing during the day.

10. Dehydration

The importance of adequate water intake for health cannot be overemphasized. It turns out that… when this is lacking… you may suffer a migraine attack.

Around a third of people who have this disorder often report dehydration as a trigger. It is not necessary to be severely dehydrated; being mildly so may be enough for an attack. The risk for dehydration increases in the presence of too much heat.

Soft drinks or soda are no substitutes to water. They not only dehydrate you further, but can also contain sweeteners, such as aspartame, which are associated with migraine.

11. Exercise

Exercise is good for health and all that, but you need to do it wisely. It is actually thought to help in fighting migraine. When you work out, your body releases natural pain relievers and you feel better.

Things can take a turn for the worse when you exercise inappropriately. For example, if you are someone who is not used to exercising regularly, you could trigger an attack if you start working out intensively all of a sudden.

Staring at a visual display unit, monitor or computer screen for extended period of time is another reason you may have migraine.

Some Risk Factors

The factors we discussed in this chapter are some of those that can cause or trigger a migraine attack. There are still some other possible triggers.

There are certain risk factors as well. As we already mentioned, women are more likely to have this primary headache disorder than men. Also, having someone in your family who has this problem means you are at a higher risk of having it.

You stand a higher chance of being able to stop migraine attacks by being familiar with some of the common triggers. This helps you to know what things or place you need to avoid.

It helps to have a personal migraine diary. You can use this to take note of what usually comes in advance of an attack. By doing this, you may be able to identify some of these common causes and triggers or something else that we did not mention here.